Paleo Diet for Athletes

By M. Usman

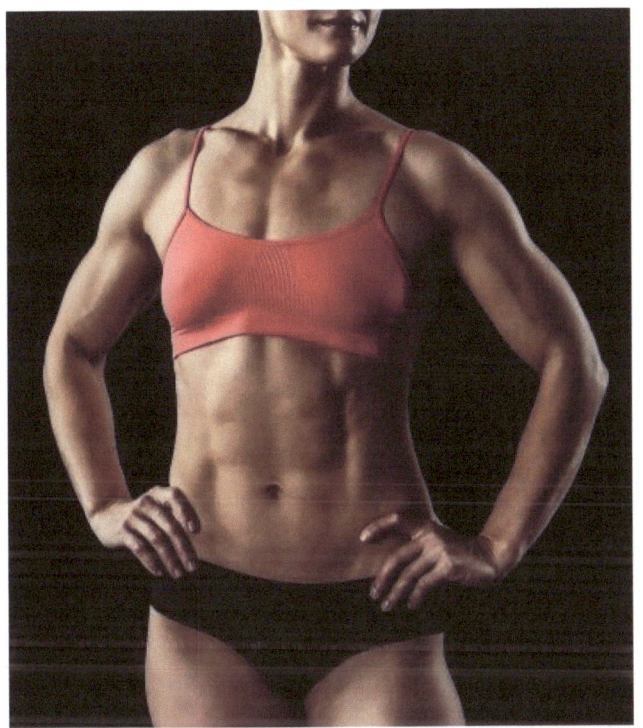

Health Learning Series
Mendon Cottage Books

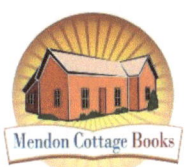

JD-Biz Publishing

Disclaimer

The information is this book is provided for informational purposes only. It is not intended to be used and medical advice or a substitute for proper medical treatment by a qualified health care provider. The information is believed to be accurate as presented based on research by the author.

The contents have not been evaluated by the U.S. Food and Drug Administration or any other Government or Health Organization and the contents in this book are not to be used to treat cure or prevent disease.

The author or publisher are not responsible for the use or safety of any diet, procedure or treatment mentioned in this book. The author or publisher is not responsible for errors or omissions that may exist.

Warning

The Book is for informational purposes only and before taking on any diet, treatment or medical procedure it is recommended to consult with your primary care provider.

Our books are available at

1. Amazon.com
2. Barnes and Noble
3. Itunes
4. Kobo
5. Smashwords
6. Google Play Books

Table of Contents

Preface

Try our diet and get leaner; try our diet and you'll lose 10 pounds in a week, try our diet and you'll never have to do cardio again; and the list goes on and on. In today's world dieting has become more of a business than a way to benefit people's lives. There are hundreds of diets out there and dozens making their way into the market, all cleverly advertised to target the core weakness of every consumer: A promise to make your life better. This is largely a hollow promise but still 'health corporations' succeed in trapping hundreds of thousands of people.

So the question arises what is so special about the Paleo diet that makes it worth trying? For starters, the Paleo diet isn't a new thing; it wasn't created a few years or decades ago by some professor in a testing lab. The Paleo diet was a result of humans' fight for survival, it was what our ancestors used to eat 10,000 years ago; right around the time when there were no grocery stores, super markets and fast-food. Eating wasn't something to do in free time; to eat one had to search for his/her food, hunt it down and cook it in/on whatever was available. Thus, Paleo is not just a diet it's a lifestyle, one which will truly make your life healthier.

The Paleo diet was just revived and popularized in the 70s by a Gastroenterologist Walter L. Voegtlin. This led to one research paper after another, one book after another being published by several doctors and nutritionists. By the 90s the Paleo diet had made its mark on the dieting market and had started to shape the dieting landscape. Practitioners started to create derivatives of the diet, synthesizing the pure Paleo meals by adding extra 'ingredients'. In this book, I will only be using pure Paleo meals as a guide to a 'better life'. This book is written keeping in mind the physical side of a healthier lifestyle. You'll see how athletes can benefit from the Paleo diet; be it swimmers, wrestlers, runners, or players of any game. The claims will be backed by scientific evidence and you'll see progress within weeks.

Getting Started

Chapter # 1: An Introduction

Who is an athlete? An athlete is anyone who takes part in sports involving strength, dexterity or endurance. Athletics include and are not limited to running, jumping, throwing, weight-lifting, baseball, basketball, shot-put, etc. To be the best athletes must eat food that enhances their physical strength and allows them to get the most out of their bodies. For this reason many professional athletes even have their own customized meal plans and personal dieticians. This is not the only reason to hire dieticians; the major reasons are the diet plans that pop out of the market every week.

Not everyone can afford this kind of help and if one can find a good, effective diet plan for him/herself there will be no need to spend thousands of extra dollars on personalized content, even by professional athletes. The Paleo diet is the answer to this question.

As stated in the preface, the Paleo diet is not just a diet but a whole lifestyle change; humans had to hunt to gather food in the Paleolithic period. Of course this can't happen nowadays due to the adequate amount of food supply we have, but followers of the diet can get involved in some sport to make up for the loss; And there you have it. The Paleo diet's the answer for every athlete out there. This diet was specifically created with physical activity at its core. This is not mandatory if you want to follow the diet but it is highly recommended if you want to reap full rewards of the regimen.

The Paleo diet, being a selective in nature places its followers within some constraints. A comprehensive list of its food items is given in the table on the next page.

Allowed	Not Allowed
Lean red meats, game meats, and organ meats	Grains & cereals
Pork	Beans
Poultry	Legumes
Fish and Shellfish	Dairy products
Eggs	Salt
Leafy and cruciferous vegetables	Refined sugar
Root vegies	Refined fats
Mushrooms	Canned or processed meat
Fruits	Fatty meats
Nuts	Bacon
Raw Honey	Soda and fruit juices

Chapter # 2: Between the lines

An athlete's first and foremost requirements are fats & proteins and lots of it. But that's not the end of it. The body must also be able to use them and not just stock them up. A very common mistake made by beginners is consuming a lot of sweets in search of energy. Sweets are simply carbohydrates; the food type restricted by the Paleo diet. Carbohydrates include candy, jams, desserts, cereals, bread and pasta. Eating carbs give you energy but this only works in the short-term. To get this concept let me take you into a little more detail.

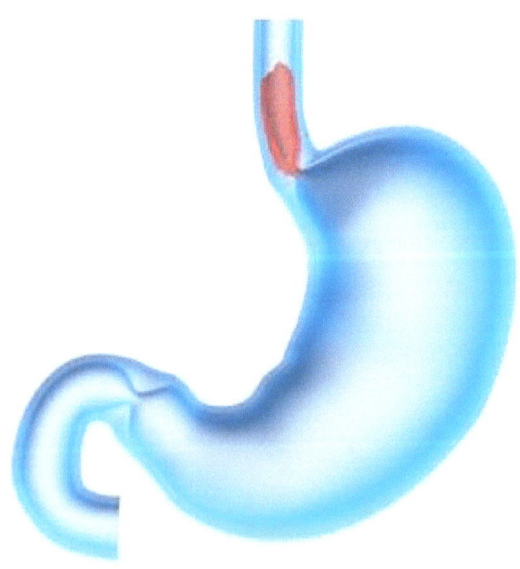

Our body's requires glucose, which is a form of sugar for energy. Glucose can be prepared in two ways; the easiest being by burning glycogen. If carbs are present your body, first they will be utilized and only then can other sources such as fats be used to manufacture glucose. Even if you consume a meal containing proteins and fats along with carbohydrates, nothing good will expectedly come out. The reason is simple; your body will first burn all the carbs and then turn to fats for fuel. So only if you limit the amount of carbs in your body, can you benefit from the Paleo diet.

Here's what happens when you stop the carb madness and switch to the Paleo diet. Firstly, your body uses carbs to produce glucose but as soon as it runs out, your body switches to fats. The process of using fats for energy is known as ketosis. Simply put, ketosis converts fats to ketone bodies which are then converted to glucose. After this process is initiated, it can take some time before your body adjusts itself to the new fuel source therefore, you may experience some headaches, fatigue and nausea. This effect only lasts for 2 weeks so it's best to give yourself a break, physically until your body adapts.

So you get the picture, don't you? Once you switch to the Paleo diet, your body will turn to fat for energy. This will result in the extra deposited fat being burned to make way for healthy muscles.

Chapter # 3: Added Benefits

When you switch to the Paleo diet, burning fat is not the only thing you benefit from. Your health takes a positive turn too. The following are some of the health benefits other than fat loss that you get from the Paleo diet:

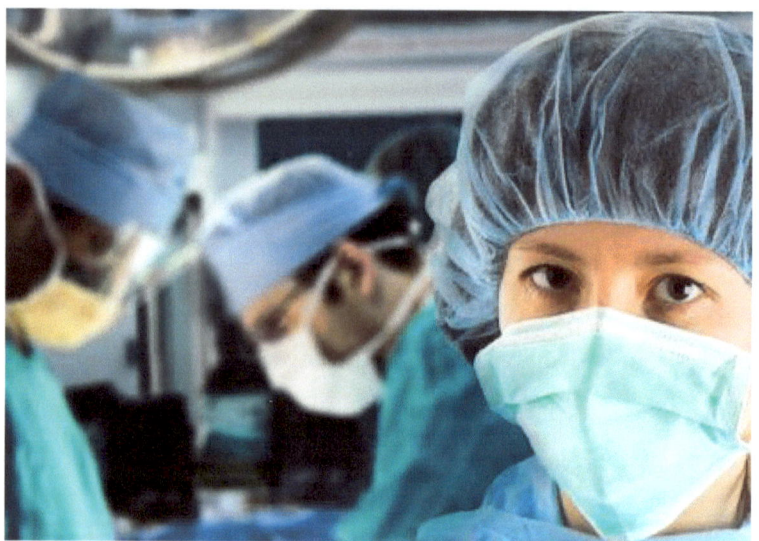

- As the Paleo diet eliminates processed foods from your diet you are protected from the numerous harmful additives, color, flavorings and who knows what else.

- Paleo diet is not just about proteins and fats. It is loaded with vegetables, nuts, berries and fruits. These food items are rich in nutrients which help in improving gut health and nutrient absorption.

- Paleo diet limits sodium intake that helps to decrease bloat, felt after eating western diet. This combined with a lot of fiber and water helps in a healthy digestive system.

- Fats and proteins in Paleo meals are very satisfying. The energy provided by proteins, fats and a few carbs is transferred in the body gradually and evenly. Therefore, blood sugar levels remain under control and energy drops are rare.

- Paleo diet provides the body with Omega-3 and 6 fatty acids in a healthy ratio help in maintaining arteries, brain function and healthy skin.

- Furthermore, the Paleo diet helps in improving sleep patterns, healthier hair, mental clarity, improved mood, and improvement in asthma condition, lower risk of heart disease, control over diabetes and reduced allergies.

Chapter # 4: Switching to the Paleo diet

All that is required to make a smooth transition to the Paleo lifestyle is a dash of determination and some guidance. The process of switching to Paleo diet is not a hard or painful one but more like a detox one. The good news for athletes is that as their diet is mostly made up of proteins and fats, this phase is very unlikely to be noticed and you'll be good to go in a week.

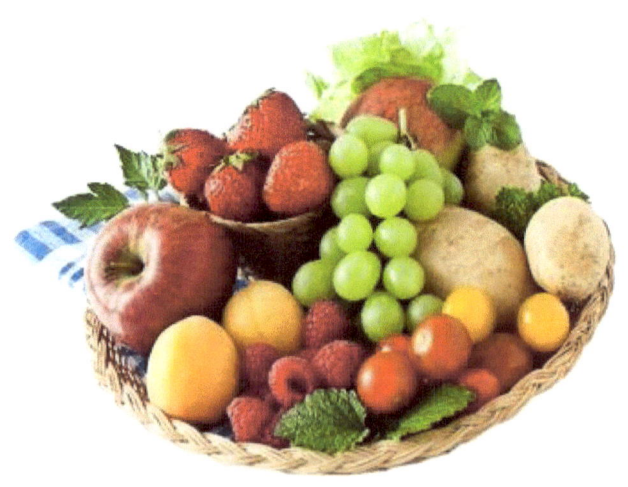

First of all, don't go cold turkey. Do everything in a managed, moderate manner. Get rid of any processed foods like rice, bread, cereal, potato chips, pasta, cakes, etc. Lower your carbohydrate intake gradually, every day for a week. Considering you consume protein on a daily basis, start adding fresh vegetables to your meals. Cook meals in corn oil, olive oil and unsaturated fats. Avoid ghee at all costs. Drink only water with lemon juice and maple syrup. Over the next week, phase out processed foods from your diet. If you must, eat whole-foods only.

After 1-2 days of switching to the Paleo diet you might notice some withdrawal symptoms, occasion energy loss. But this only means that the Paleo diet is working. Your body is switching to fats for fuel and is discarding carbs. Very often you will get the temptation to eat something sweet; if you do drink some herbal tea.

After 1 week, you would notice that something different is happening, something soothing; your energy's back and this time it stays constant throughout the course of the day. Your craving for synthesized food diminishes.

Congratulations, your body is now ready for the Paleo diet.

Paleo Specifics

Chapter # 5: Importance of BCAAs

Ever wondered what muscle proteins are made up of? The answer is BCAAs. BCAAs or Branched chain amino acids are the core of our muscles. Amino acids like leucine, valine and isoleucine make up BCAAs but the detail is not necessary. So what is so special about these amino acids? These amino acids cannot be manufactured inside the human body. But still our body needs them and only way to acquire them is by eating food items that do. These food items include lean meat, beef, chicken and turkey. As meat and its variants make up a huge part of the Paleo diet, followers of the diet have no trouble obtaining BCAAs.

BCAAs are important for everyone but they hold a special importance when it comes to athletes. Here's why:

- **They play a huge role in building muscles in your body:**
  During physical work-outs you require a lot of energy as your metabolism rates reaches the sky. Firstly, carbs stored in muscles are called up for the task, as soon as they run out BCAAs replace carbs as the fuel. BCAAs are then converted to glucose. Thus, a diet rich in BCAAs would help prevent extra muscle breakdown. As BCAAs are the building blocks of proteins, it is quite clear that consuming a diet rich in them would aid in muscle growth.
  When under stress a hormone, cortisol is released that breaks down proteins for energy. BCAAs promote the release of a growth stimulating hormone that increases muscle mass, i.e. testosterone. The gain in mass of your body will be judged by the ratio between

the two hormones. Higher testosterone levels will mean your muscle mass will increase whereas lower would result in loss. Research has shown that BCAAs help bring hormone imbalances under control. A report was published in "Chinese general of physiology", in which the effects of "BA or BCAA drink on hormone changes after strenuous exercise were studied in comparison to a placebo drink (PL). According to the report the ratio between the two hormones after 120 minutes was higher in BA trial as compared to the PA one. This shows that BCAAs trigger anabolic response during recovery.

Therefore, the Paleo diet is very important for athletes as muscle is the true power house of a sportsman.

- **They help the body loose unwanted fat:**

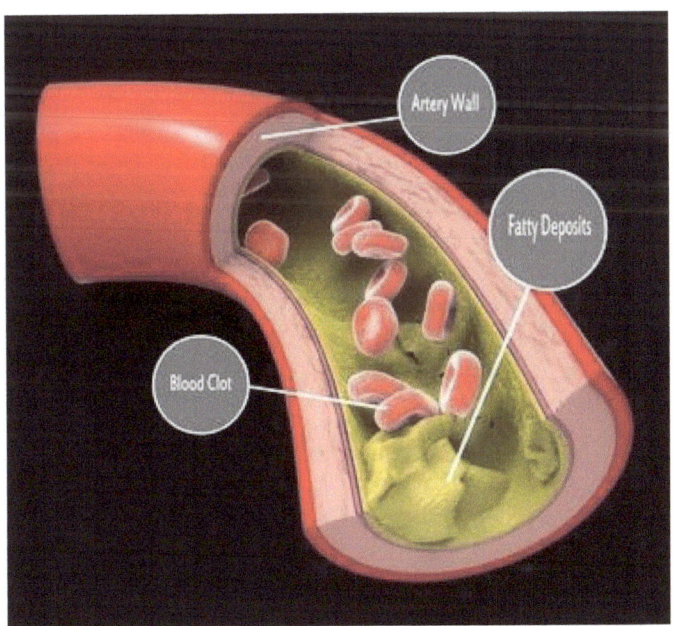

A report published by the "American journal of nutrition" stated that after carrying out trials on 4000 volunteers it was found that obesity and BCAA intake was inversely proportional. There was a lower prevalence of obesity in all those who were on BCAA supplements as compared to those who were no. Thus, the body gets a definitive posture and figure, a necessity for every athlete.

- **An increase in stamina and decrease in muscle pains:**

  A research carried out by Sacred Heart University showed that BCCA supplementation decreased muscle damages and pains after severe workouts. There were fewer complains about muscle soreness and inflammations. Participants are able to last longer in exercises and able to do more intensive workouts. This research was carried out on middle aged, untrained men. Just imagine what effect BCCA would have on professional athletes.

- **Health brain performance:**

  This one's not really for the athletes but it's always good to know something's got your back during competitions and pressurizing moments. It has been found that BCAAs increase reaction times and improve the brain's cerebral abilities. They also help in alleviating bad moods and tensions.

Chapter # 6: Importance of Simple Carbs

After intense physical workout your body needs some time to recover. Your energy stores take a hit and your muscles break down. Therefore, it is important to re-fuel your body with the right type and amounts of food types, at the right time. Even though, the Paleo diet has a strict policy about carbs; simple carbs are not harmful to the body and when taken in the right amount, are valuable.

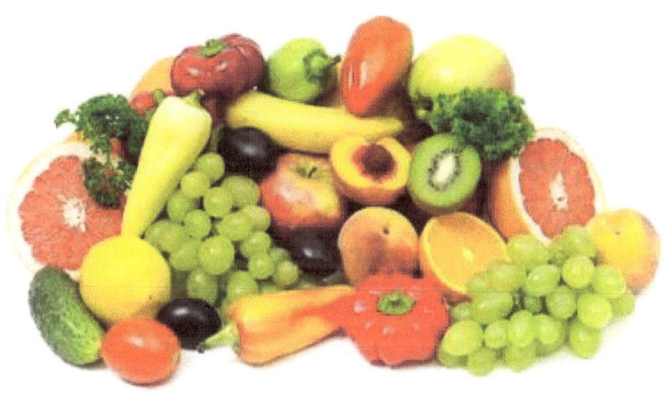

What is the difference between simple carbs and complex carbs? There are is a huge difference between simple and complex carbs. Glucose and fructose are a few sugars included in the simple carb group. We acquire them from fruits. Glucose is what our body ultimately needs as fuel and requires no further metabolism. As simple carbs provide this, there is no need for any further processing and the carbs can quickly be absorbed into the blood, where they can be directly used as fuel. This is not the case with complex carbs; Complex carbs have a complicated structure and require further break down to be used as fuel. Complex carbs are found in cereals and starch. They include sugars like sucrose. Thus, it takes some time for the complex carbs to settle in and this is not what your body needs after an intense workout.

During workouts, your body burns glycogen in your muscles to provide instant energy. After these stores are depleted, you can't work out any more and you need some quick energy boost. This is where simple carbs come in; they provide a quick energy boost to restore your lost energy. When you consume simple carbs, your body releases insulin to metabolize these carbs, converting them into glycogen. In addition they start the process of synthesizing body proteins, which help increase muscle mass. Furthermore, insulin helps in neutralizing the effect of another hormone called cortisol. This hormone is the main culprit behind muscle loss and breakdown. Insulin alleviates this hormone and thus prevents further muscle loss. But this does not mean that, the more insulin there is the more muscle you build. If there is excess of sugars in your body, the insulin can work against you. If there is too much sugar in your post workout meal, the insulin would start to decrease this sugar, leading to a decrease in muscle mass. It would convert this sugar into fat and this would run water over all your work outs and strict diet plans.

To tackle these effects, you should follow some simple guidelines:

- Consume these carbs 20-30 minutes after your workout.

- Consume about 15-20 grams of simple carbs during you post-workout sessions. This amount is best for these carbs to be converted into sugar. If you consume more carbs, the insulin would start converting them into fats rather than proteins.

So you see that even though simple carbs of aren't allowed by the Paleo regimen, you should make an exception for simple carbs as they are very beneficial and do not hinder the progress made by the Paleo diet in any way.

Specific recipes on post-workout meals are given in the next section.

Diet Plan

Chapter # 7: Basic Paleo Plan

Paleo diet is very effective in burning unnecessary fat off you and keeping it off. To get every possible benefit from the Paleo diet, you must follow some general rules. Specific recipes are given in later chapters.

- Consume 4-8 ounces of lean meat, chicken, turkey or seafood.

- Add servings of colored vegetables either steamed or raw, to your food.

- Round up your meal with a handful of unsalted nuts like almonds, walnuts and peanuts.

Consume 2-3 meals like this per day, follow these rules for 30 days and you'll see how effectively Paleo diet keeps unwanted bulk off.

The needs of athletes vary depending on the level of activity and the type of sport. Despite this, there are a few major things that all these athletes share and must focus on them in order to perform in their sports respectively:

- Optimizing performance

- Improving recovery

Good news, as the Paleo diet provides the perfect solution for both improving performance and recovery times. Lean proteins enhance your performance and because of huge quantity of Branched chain amino acids in your diet your body recovers rapidly after a heavy workout. Therefore, this proves to be excellent for both strength as well as endurance athletes.

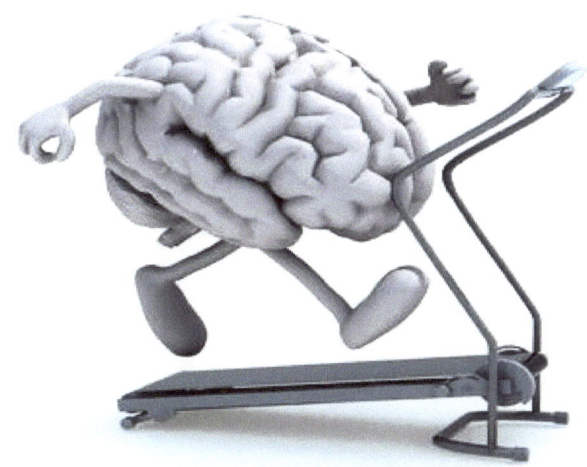

The next customization is based on the type of sport you play. High intensity aerobic, anaerobic (soccer, martial arts, boxing) and sprinters should take advantage of the short time after training when the body recovers. Carbs such as sweet potatoes, fruits and yams can prove very helpful in repairing damaged muscle tissues and replenishing glycogen supplies to the muscles if consumed within 40 minutes of workout/training. The amount of carbs you consume will be dependent on your body's size and the intensity of your training. The bigger you are the harder you must train and therefore, you require a bigger dose of carbohydrates to optimize recovery. For sprinters and other endurance athletes, a diet of lean proteins and low carb vegetables along with good fats is ideal.

Eating low carb foods along with regular Paleo ones is quite a good combo as it proves very effective with field athletes, Olympic weight lifters and others who rely on their strength, stamina and low body fat during a competition.

For best possible results consume one gram of protein for every pound in your body.

Chapter # 8: Pre-workout meals

When preparing your pre-workout meal, be sure to go after something that produces energy, provides protein and can be made quickly. Here are few recipes that ought to do it:

- **Peaches and brazil nuts:**

  Pick up a peach and a handful of Brazil nuts (around six) on the way to the gym or field. Brazil nuts are the key here. They provide you with a substantial amount of calories and unsaturated fats; this gives you a quick boost ideal for a hard workout. These nuts also incorporate trace mineral, selenium; research has shown that it can increase testosterone levels. The peach provides much needed sugar that can be used as a quick power source in intensive workouts.

- **Turkey and avocado:**

  While cooking breakfast, throw in some slices of turkey; wrap them up in a foil and just an hour before work-out take them out. Slice up a fresh avocado and there you have it, in less than 5 minutes you have yourself a snack filled with proteins and energy.

- **Chicken and Sweet potato:**

  If you are cooking chicken for dinner, make sure you add a few extra pieces to save up for the workout. Six ounces of chicken for workout will be ideal. This will provide you will the right amount of protein for harder workouts. Pick-up a sweet potato as it is a source of natural carbohydrates. It would provide an excellent energy boost to your body.

- **Apple, hardboiled eggs and a few blueberries:**

This may sound like a smorgasbord of a lot of Paleo meals but if you would try it, you would come to know its nutritious benefits. This random snack would provide you with proteins, a good supply of fats and fructose that would give you the benefit of slow as well as fast burning energy.

- **Orange with some coconut oil:**

This one's for all those in a hurry. Get an orange along with two teaspoons of coconut oil and some sugarless coffee. This will allow you to do at least 30 minutes of high intensity training and 1 hour of moderate one. There will also be a mental kick after you eat these foods that will work as motivation for the workout.

- **Almont infused shake:**

Take two scoops of whey protein (approximately 35 grams) and then a cup of sugar free vanilla almond milk. If you can, mix a teaspoon of natural honey and some almond butter. And there you have it; a great tasting shake. The shake is loaded with goodness or proteins, good fats and simple carbs from honey. This can be prepared in less than 2 minutes so it's great for a quick takeout. Be sure to have it 45 minutes prior to your training. This will give you adequate time to digest it and the shake to do provide you with an energy spike.

Chapter # 9: Post-workout meals

Remember, post-workout snacks should be small, energizing and easy to prepare.

- It's best to start out with an energizing protein shake. Mix two glasses of raw milk, 2 egg yolks, a banana and almonds in a blender. This will provide you with an immediate energy boost and you will feel refreshed.

- Mix half a cup of coconut milk, some cashew butter, half a banana, two dried dates, one tablespoon maple syrup and ice cubes as required. Add this to a blender and mix until you feel it's ready.

- Mix one cup of sugarless pineapple juice (best if natural) with one cup of coconut milk, half a cup of lime juice and a banana. Add ice cubes and blend to your liking.

- Mix one cup of fresh cherries, 2 tablespoon sugarless cocoa powder, a cup of almond milk and half a banana. Sprinkle with coconut shavings. Add a few ice cubes and blend to your liking.

- Mix a cup of coconut cream, a tablespoon of cocoa powder, 8 -10 mint leaves, and a tablespoon of coconut syrup. Add crushed ice and blend to your liking.

- Eat 7-8 raisins as they help in restoring the body's alkalinity and continue to help the body recover for the next repetitions.

- Foods rich in simple carbs such as avocados, dates, cinnamon, coconut and multi-colored berries.

- A lot of water or 300 – 400 ml of orange juice. You will immediately feel refreshed (it's no secret).

- If you work out at home or someplace close to your house; you can try 12 ounces of raw beef with some mustard and a cup of sweet potatoes (mashed) with butter.

- Poach a salmon; add half a cup of honey dew and some blueberries.

- Grilled salmon with olive oil and cinnamon.

- Asparagus, mushroom, coconut milk and bamboo shoot curry.

Chapter # 10: Breakfast Recipes

1. **Almond Flour Muffins:** **(makes 4 muffins)**

   Take four ounces of almond flour and empty in a medium sized bowl. Add a quarter teaspoon of baking soda into the bowl. Take a large bowl and scramble two eggs, one tablespoon honey and half tablespoon apple vinegar. Transfer the contents of the medium sized bowl into the large one and mix them well. Scoop quarter cup of batter into a muffin pan; bake at 350 degrees for 20 minutes. Take them out when the edges are brown and cool them for half an hour. Serve with jam or butter.

2. **Green eggs:**

   Take four eggs, three kale leaves (untrimmed) , and a pinch of sea salt in a blender. Blend until the mixture is lump free. Heat some oil in a pan and pour the contents of the blender on it. Cook the mixture for some time and then scramble. Keep cooking until you achieve your desired doneness.

3. **Granola:** **(serves 12)**

   Place 10 – 15 almonds, 10 macadamia nuts, and one cup pumpkin seeds in a large bowl half filled with water. Place one cup raisins in a bowl half filled with water. Let the nuts and raisins soak overnight. Puree the raisins along with their soaking until smooth. Use a metal strainer to drain and rinse the nuts and seeds in the first bowl. Add these nuts and seeds to pureed raisins. Use a food processor or otherwise, to coarsely chop this mixture. Finally, add one tablespoon vanilla extract, half tablespoon cinnamon and a pinch of sea salt. Mix these contents briefly. Transfer this mixture onto 2-3 parchment lined sheets. Place in an oven at 135 degrees for 24 hours. If you need it right away, bake it at 250 for 45 minutes. Add some coconut shavings and serve.

4. **Chocolate chip scones:** **(makes 8 scones)**

Add half a cup of coconut flour, quarter teaspoon sea salt and baking soda of the same amount into a food processor. Pulse in quarter cup of vegan shortening, quarter cup of honey and four eggs. Scoop the batter onto a baking sheet and bake at 350 degrees for 15 minutes. Cool them down and serve.

Chapter # 11: Lunch Recipes

1. **Green Chicken soup:**

   Add two quarts of chicken stock in a soup pot. Reserve two cups of stock and place the pot over medium heat. Take the reserved stock and blend it with one bunch chopped kale until it turns lump free and creamy. Pour this mixture into the chicken stock pot. Take 3 carrots, slice them and add them to the pot. If you have some shiitake mushrooms, toss some of them too.

2. **Asparagus Basil Salad:**

   Take one pound of asparagus and steam it for 7 minutes. Chop 2-3 tomatoes, an avocado and some basil leaves. Add these and the asparagus to a large bowl. Add quarter a cup of olive oil, two teaspoons of lemon juice and some mustard into the bowl. Sprinkle with pepper and salt.

3. **Baked Mustard Lime chicken:**

   Take half a cup of lime juice, some fresh cilantro, quarter cup of mustard, one tablespoon of olive oil, chili, salt, pepper and mix it in a food processor until all the ingredients are well combined. Take one pound of boneless chicken breast and place it in a 7 x 11 baking disk. Pour marinade over the chicken and refrigerate it for 15 minutes. Take the chicken out and bake it at 350 for 20 minutes.

Chapter # 12: Dinner Recipes

1. **Green chili turkey burgers:**

   In a medium sized bowl mix 2 cans of diced chilies, a pound of ground turkey, one cup of finely chopped cilantro, onion, two teaspoons of cumin, some chili powder and salt. Form into burgers and grill.

2. **Baked chicken meatballs:**

   Preheat your oven at 350 degrees. Take a cup of chopped zucchini, carrots, half a cup of parsley, and 3 cloves of garlic; add these to a food processor. Add quarter cup of almond flour, an egg, and one pound of boneless chicken breasts into the food processor. Add salt and chili powder and mix thoroughly. Drop balls of this chicken mixture onto a baking sheet and bake these for 20 minutes.

3. **Fish sticks:**

   Rinse fresh fillets of cod, snapper or tilapia in cold water and set on plate. Cut it into 1 by 5 inches pieces; remove any bones you find in this process. Place 2 scrambled eggs in a plate. Place one cup of almond flour in another plate. First, dip the fish into the eggs and then flour; now place it in another plate. Add 3 -4 tablespoons of olive oil in a large skillet. Heat the oil on medium heat. Place the fish sticks in the pan one by one, making sure they have some space between them. Cook them for a few minutes and then take them out on a paper towel. Serve with apple sauce, if available.

4. **Rosemary Lemon chicken:**

Take a medium bowl; pour two tablespoons of olive oil, quarter cup of lemon juice, two cloves of garlic, quarter cup of rosemary, and half a tablespoon of salt into it. Rinse one pound of chicken breasts (boneless) and place them into a 7x11 baking dish. Cover the chicken and refrigerate for 30 minutes. Heat and cook the chicken for 8-10 minutes per side. Cook for a longer time if it's not cooked in the center.

5. **Curried Shrimp:**

Pour 4 tablespoons of olive oil in a large saucepan. Take four cloves of garlic, a medium sized onion and put over low heat until they become tender. Add half a cup of tomatoes, two teaspoons of ginger and half a tablespoon of cumin, turmeric and coriander. Let this simmer for about 5 minutes. Place a shrimp in this simmering sauce and cool for another 10 minutes. Stir in some cilantro. After the shrimp is fully cooked, take it out and add three tablespoons of lime juice.

Conclusion

By now, it would be quite clear that the Paleo diet is not just some diet for losing weight but a solid, healthy solution for athletes too. Athletes and sportsmen can cut down extra fat in their bodies, build a lot of muscles and improve their performance on field just by following the incredible Paleo diet. So what are you waiting for? Switch to a better lifestyle, switch to the Paleo diet.

Author Bio

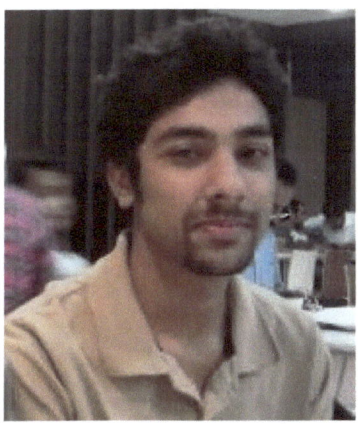

Muhammad Usman is a distinguished medical graduate of Allama iqbal medical college (AIMC). He is a professional writer who has been in the field for more than 4 years. During this time he has produced 10,000+ articles, blogs and eBooks on various niches related to diseases, health, fitness, nutrition and well-being. He is a regular contributor to several journals related to medicine and surgery. He is the editor of several journals and newspapers.

References

1. Walter Voegtlin: The Stone age diet based on in-depth study of Human ecology and diet of man (1975) – CHAPTER 15: A 20th Century Stone age diet (http://www.mitodascalorias.com/wp-content/uploads/2013/06/Voegtlin_1975_The_Stone_Age_Diet.pdf)

2. Wikipedia's definition of Paleolithic diet (http://en.wikipedia.org/wiki/Paleolithic_diet)

3. Walter Voegtlin: The Stone age diet based on in-depth study of Human ecology and diet of man (1975) (http://www.mitodascalorias.com/wp-content/uploads/2013/06/Voegtlin_1975_The_Stone_Age_Diet.pdf)

4. Boyd Eaton, Loren Cordain, Staffan Lindeberg: Evolutionary Health Promotions: A consideration of common counterarguments. December, 2001. (http://thepaleodiet.com/wp-content/uploads/2012/04/Counter-Arguments-Paper.pdf)

5. Boyd Eaton: Paleolithic nutrition – A consideration of its nature and current implications 1985 (http://www.ncbi.nlm.nih.gov/pubmed/2981409?dopt=Abstract)

6. Gary Foster et al. A randomized trial of a Low Carbohydrate diet for Obesity.

(http://inspire.stat.ucla.edu/unit_15/NEJM2082.pdf)

7. Staffan Lindeberg et al. Apparent absence of stroke and ischaemic heart disease in a traditional Melanesian island: a clinical study in Kitava. (http://onlinelibrary.wiley.com/doi/10.1111/j.1365-2796.1993.tb00986.x/abstract;jsessionid=7F1EEC9B23FCAD9333A2D12078313A4C.d02t01)

8. Loren Cordain and John Friel: The Paleo diet for athletes. (http://www.trainingbible.com/pdf/Paleo_for_Athletes_Cliff_Notes.pdf)

9. Dr. John McDougall: The Starch Solution (http://www.drmcdougall.com/store_starch_solution.html)

10. Dr. Denis Murphy: People, plants and genes – The Story of Crops and Humanity. (http://www.oxfordscholarship.com/view/10.1093/acprof:oso/9780199207145.001.0001/acprof-9780199207145)

11. Katherine Milton: Hunter-gatherer diets – a different perspective (http://ajcn.nutrition.org/content/71/3/665.long)

12. Alexander Strohle et al.: Carbohydrates and the diet-atherosclerosis connection--more between earth and heaven. Comment on the article "The atherogenic potential of dietary carbohydrate". (http://scholar.qsensei.com/content/1321gb

http://www.ncbi.nlm.nih.gov/pubmed/16997359)

13. US. News and World Reports 2012 – Best overall diets
    (http://health.usnews.com/best-diet/best-overall-diets)

Check out some of the other JD-Biz Publishing books

Gardening Series on Amazon

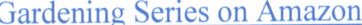

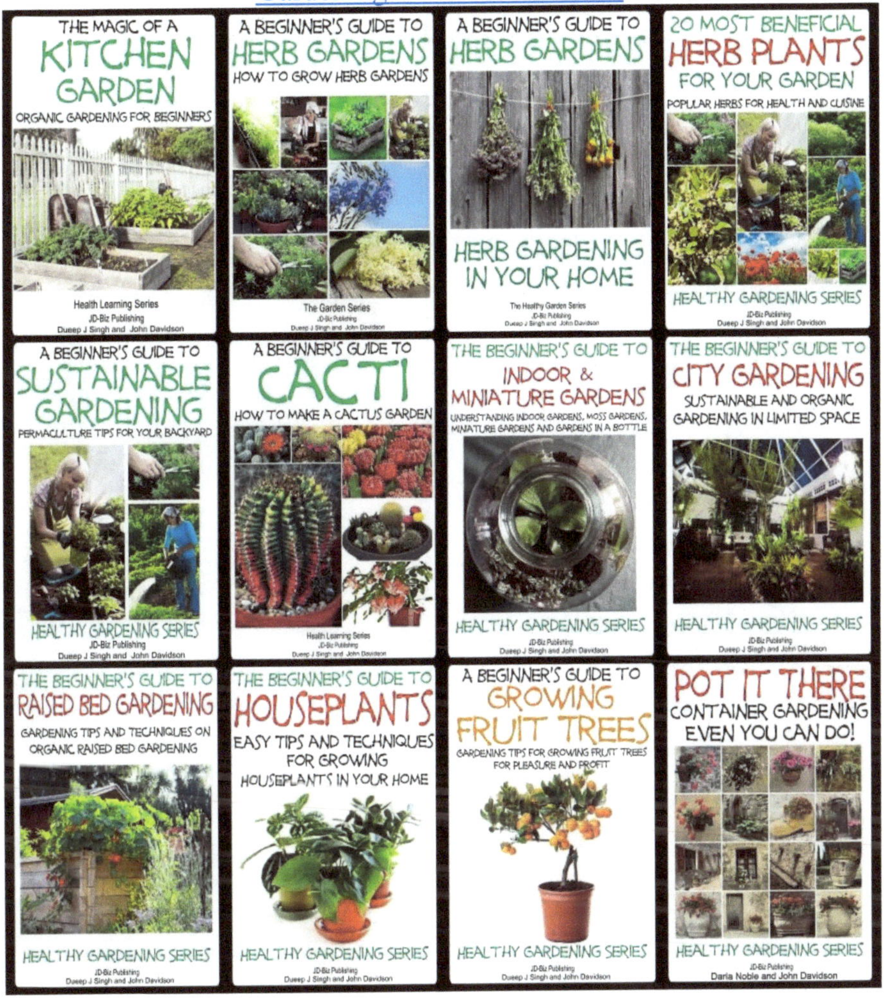

Download Free Books!
http://MendonCottageBooks.com

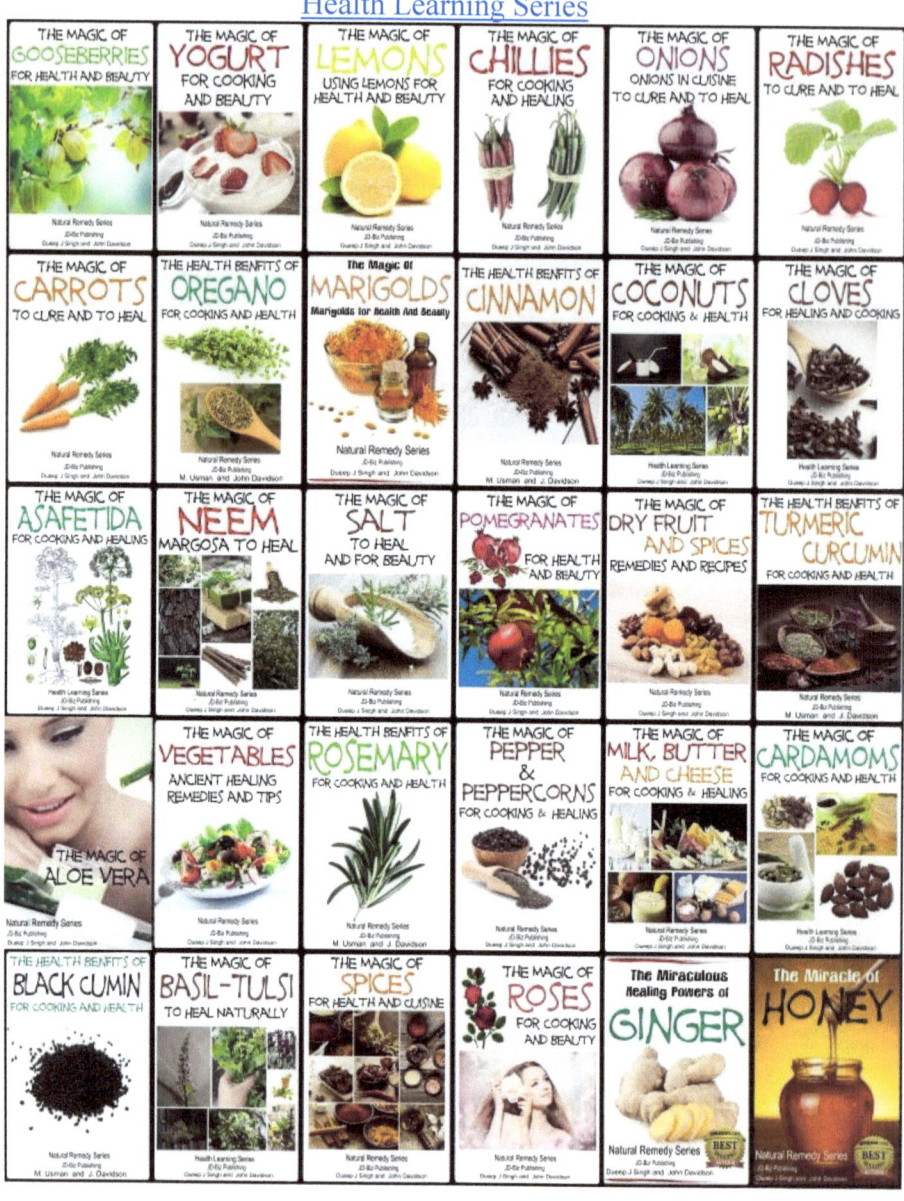

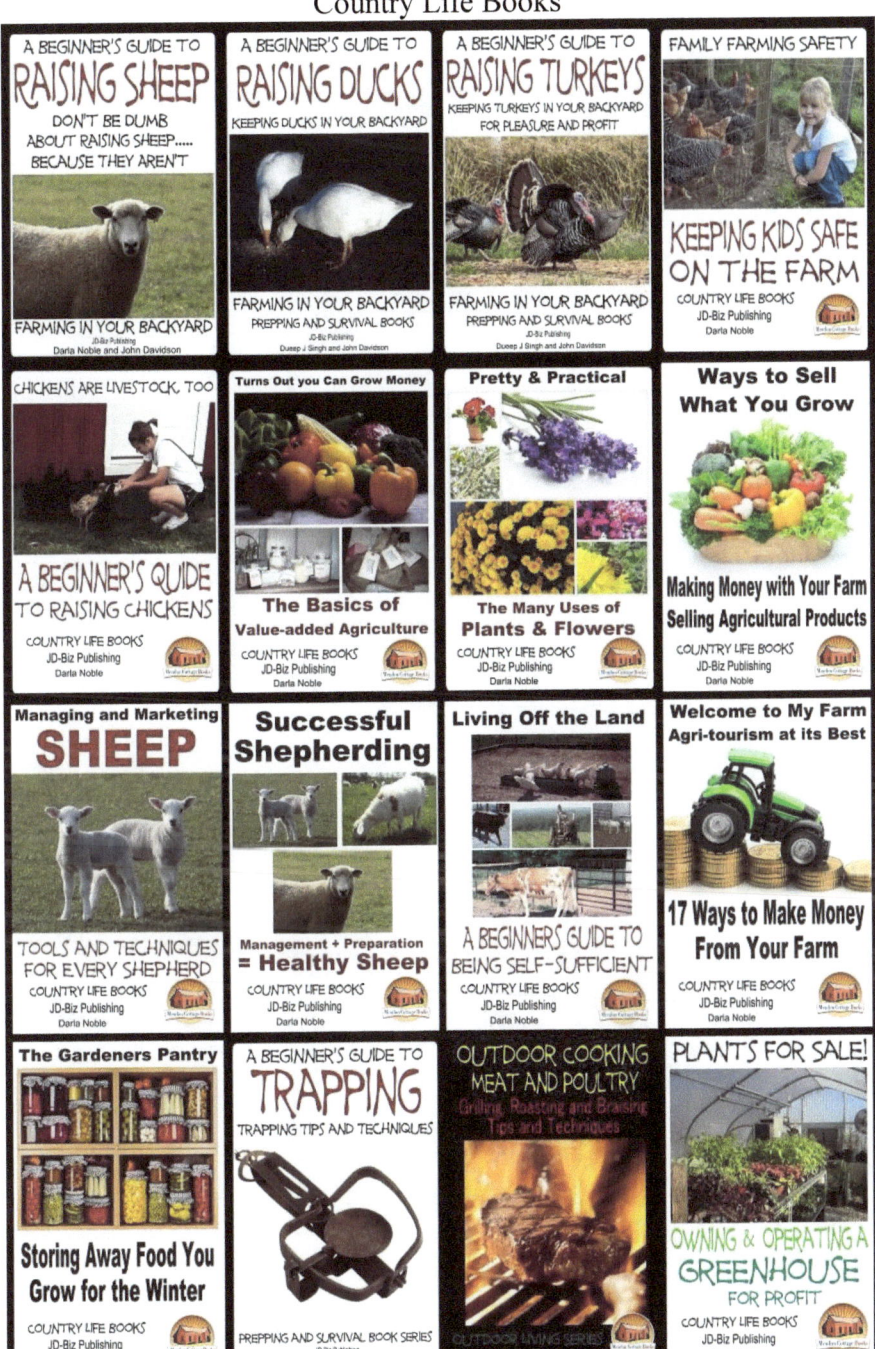

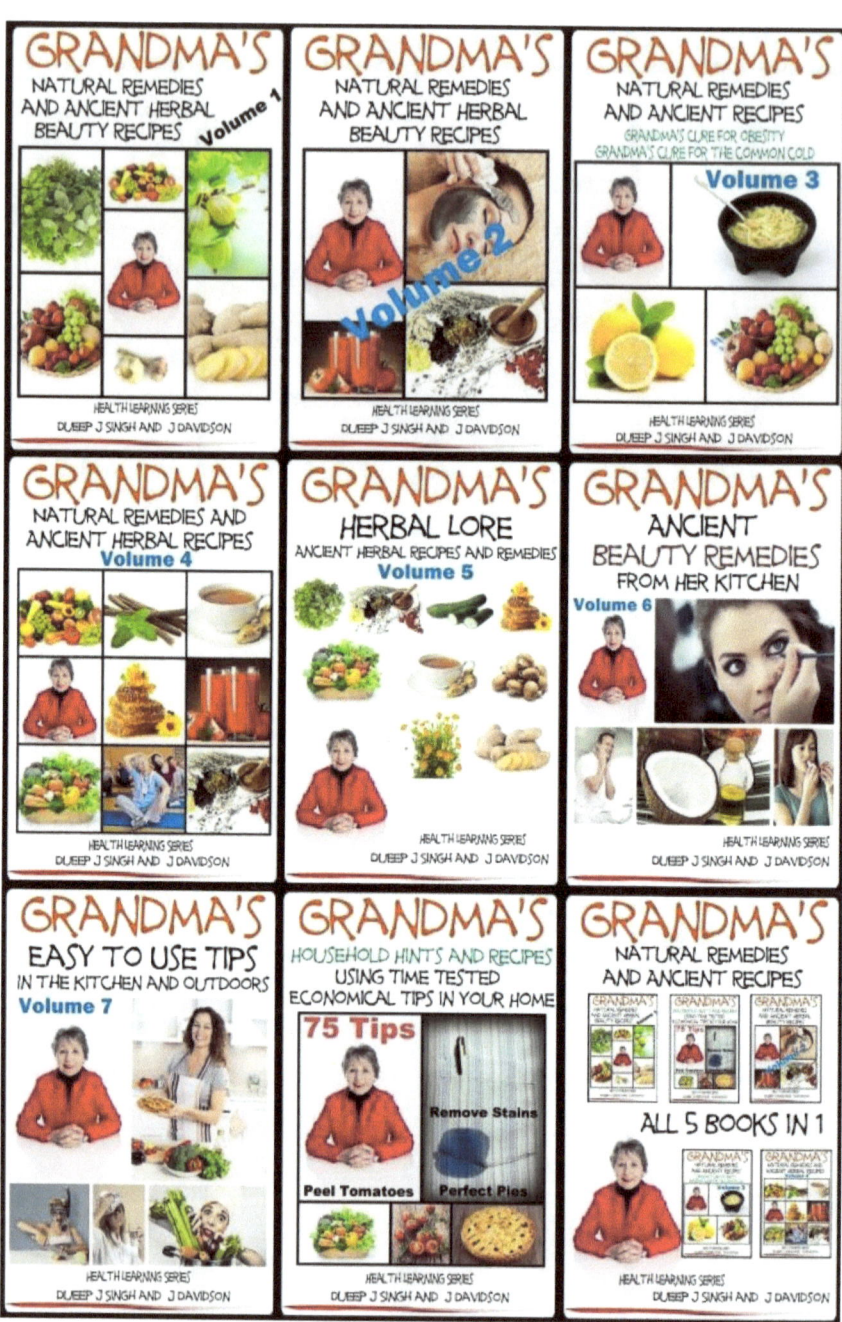

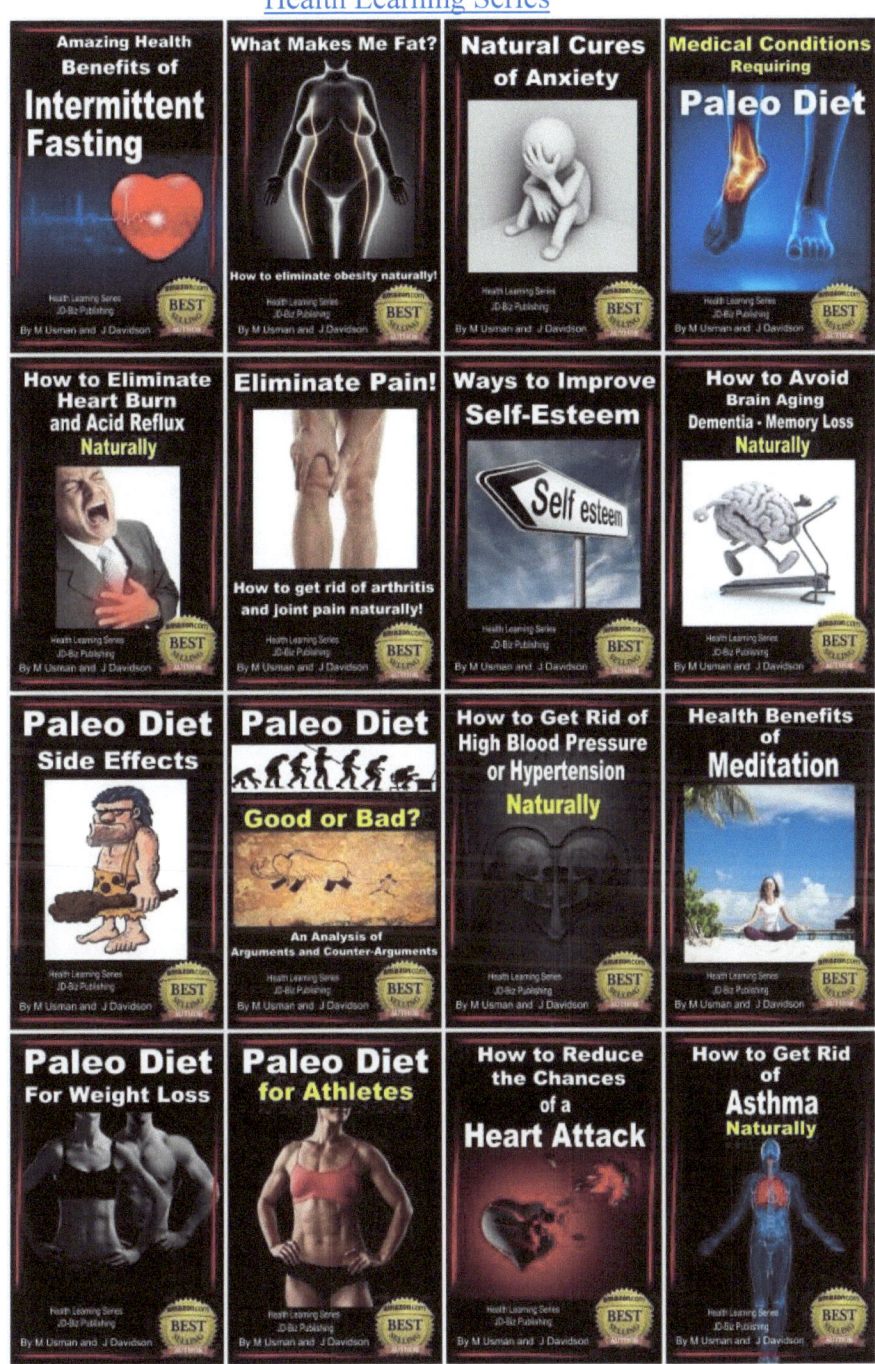

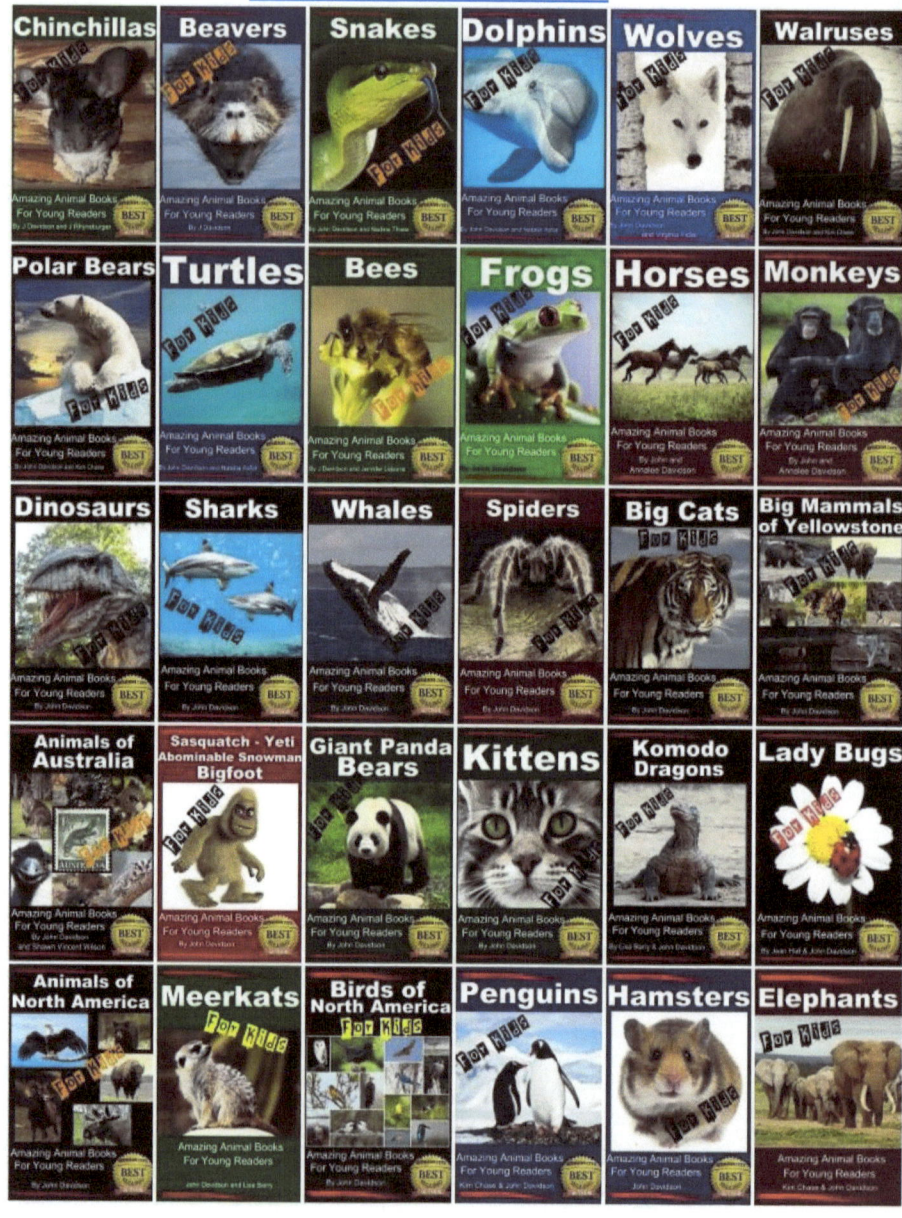

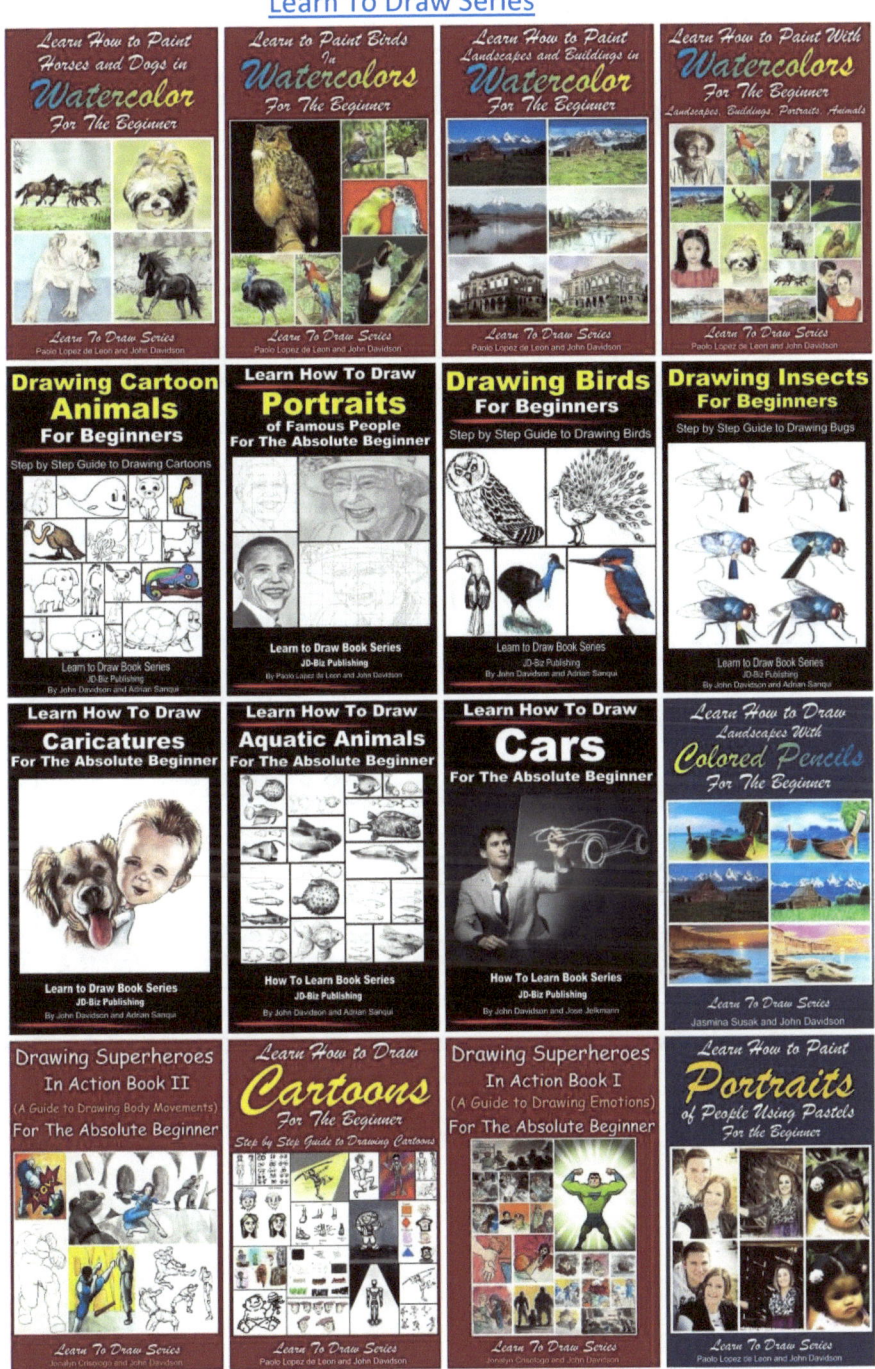

How to Build and Plan Books

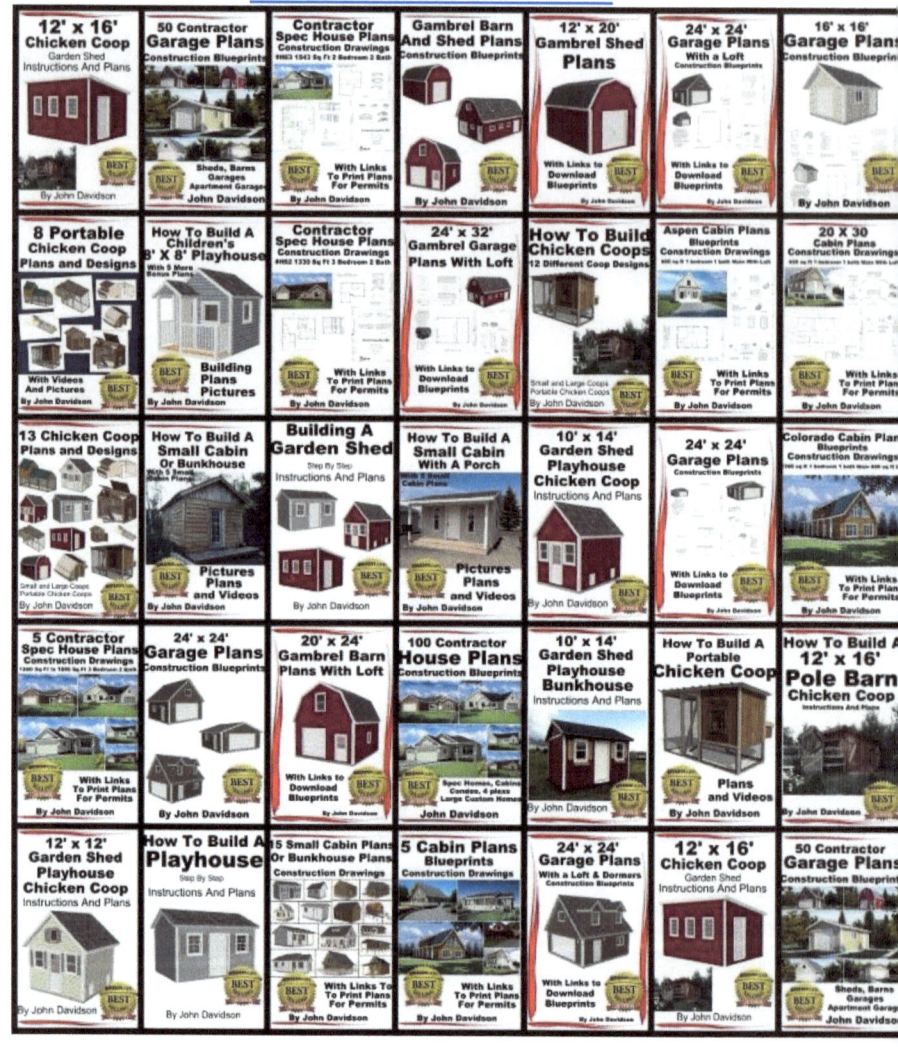

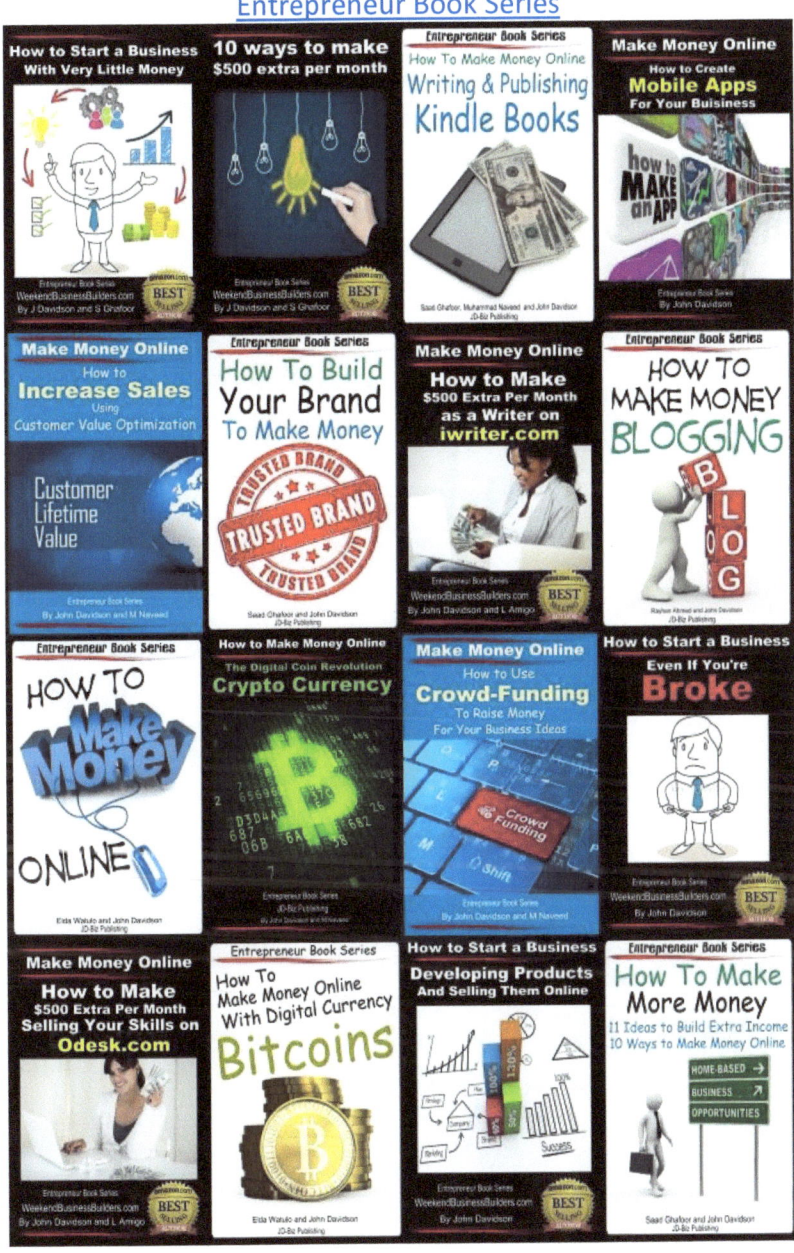

Our books are available at

1. [Amazon.com](#)
2. [Barnes and Noble](#)
3. [Itunes](#)
4. [Kobo](#)
5. [Smashwords](#)
6. [Google Play Books](#)

Download Free Books!
http://MendonCottageBooks.com

Publisher

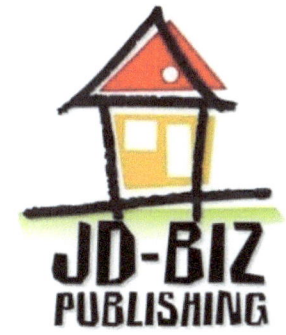

JD-Biz Corp

P O Box 374

Mendon, Utah 84325

http://www.jd-biz.com/

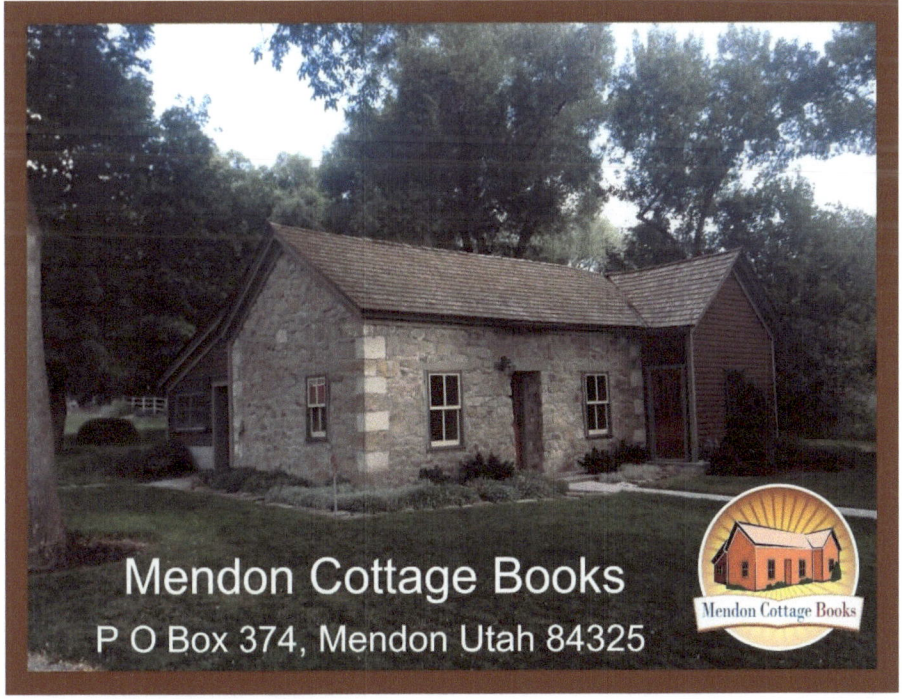

Mendon Cottage Books

P O Box 374, Mendon Utah 84325